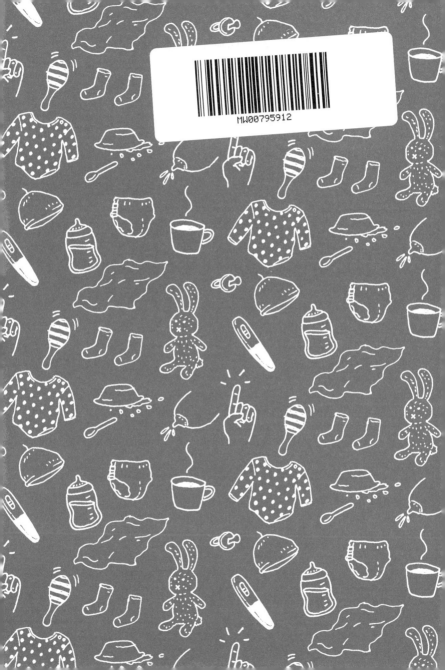

MW00795912

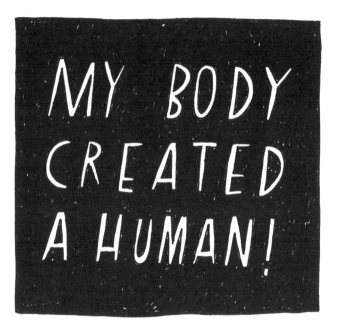

MY BODY CREATED A HUMAN!

A Love Story

Emma Ahlqvist

Princeton Architectural Press · New York

1.
There is a baby inside
of me.

I HAVE
A BABY
IN MY
BELLY!!

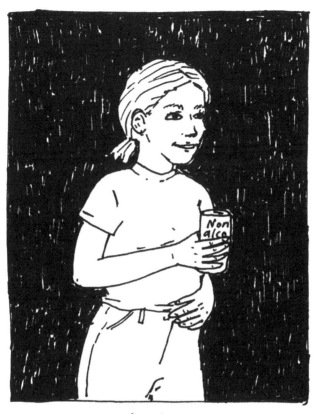

It's exciting to have this secret.

I hope that no one has realized
that I'm drinking nonalcoholic beer.

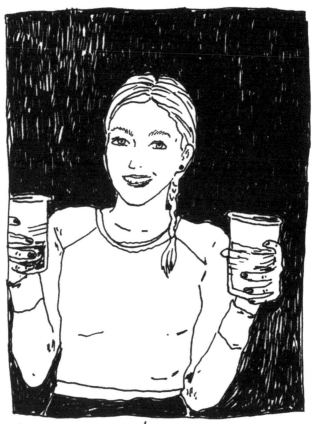

I wish I had an excuse not to go clubbing.

I spent a lot of my twenties going out, but now I'm ready for a change.

For so long, I've been preparing —
waiting to be ready.

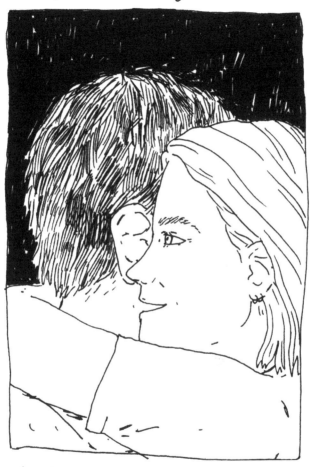

And now, I guess I am.

As soon as we decide to try, I feel desperate to get pregnant.

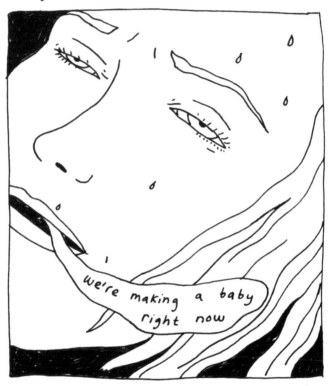

Is it weird that we both get turned on thinking about it?

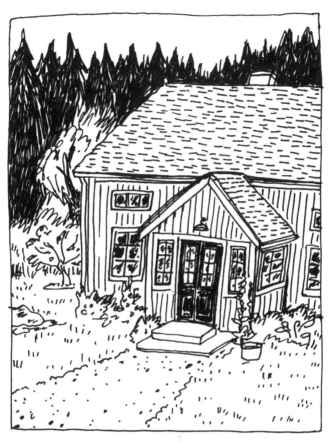

I had always imagined we'd move out of the city before having children.

Instead we live in an apartment in Edinburgh, and I'm excited about bringing up a kid wherever we are.

BABY

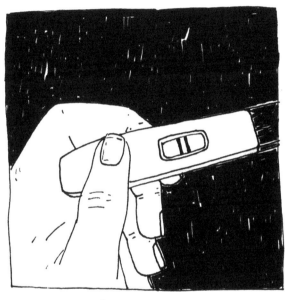

I'm used to trying to control everything in my life, and it is scary that I can't control this.

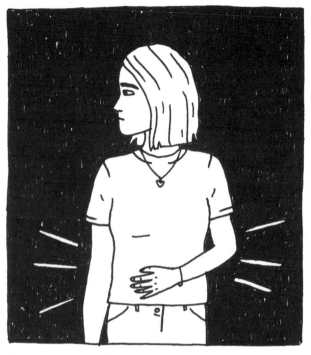

I want to tell everyone early, but it feels like I'm not allowed.

If I have a miscarriage, I think that I will want to talk about that too.

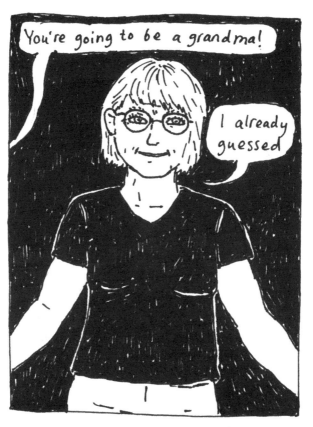

How is it that mothers always know?

Every time I wake up, I'm
shocked to remember that
I'm pregnant.

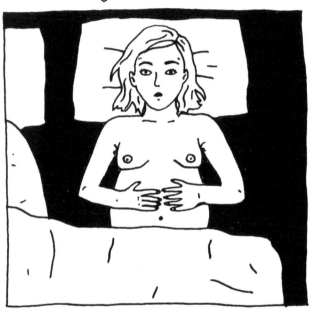

When I'm awake, I can't
stop thinking about my
pregnancy.

I feel disappointed with
my body when I hear pregnant
women saying they feel great.

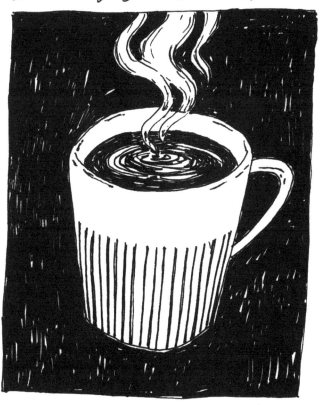

Coffee suddenly tastes like
poison, and I have constant
heartburn.

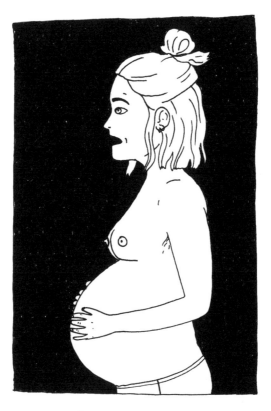

Sometimes I panic because I've forgotten that I'm making a baby, then I remember that my body is doing it all for me.

Sometimes we talk about
what will change.

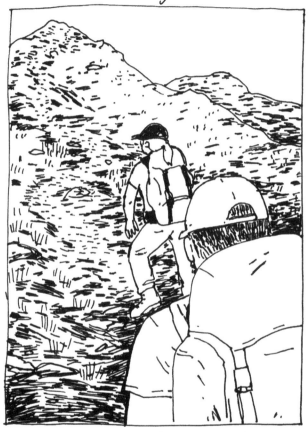

Will we still be able to do
the things we love once we
have a child?

Usually, I put a lot of pressure on myself to be a successful person. Now, I let myself do less, and it feels good.

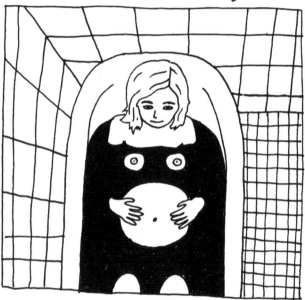

After all, I'm constantly working on creating a human.

I have always had small breasts,
but now they feel huge. It reminds
me of being a teenager and growing
breasts for the first time.

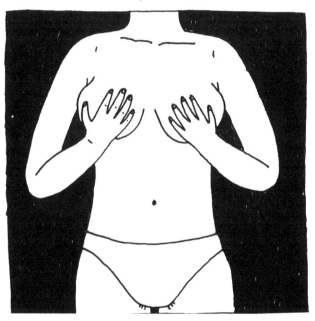

I like to hold them and feel
their weight in my hands.

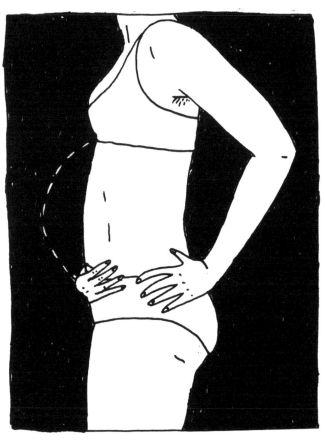

When I look back at my first
pregnancy photo, I laugh at how
I thought I looked so pregnant.

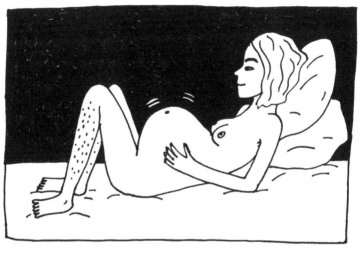

I don't want to see friends or go
out. I just want to lie in my bed
and feel the baby move in my belly.

How will I manage to go through labor when I'm so exhausted all the time?

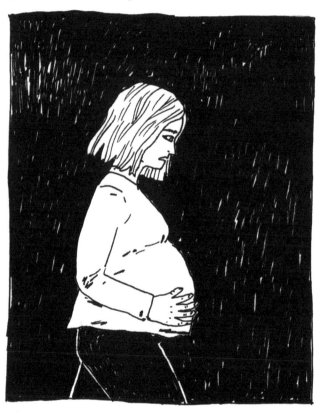

I'm trying to remember I still have that pregnancy glow.

But being pregnant has given me a new sense of purpose, even if I'm too tired to do much.

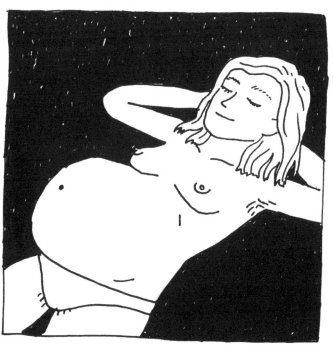

I feel so special, even if all of our mothers have already done this thing.

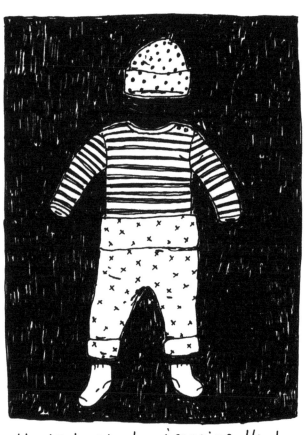

It is hard to imagine that there is a little person inside of me.

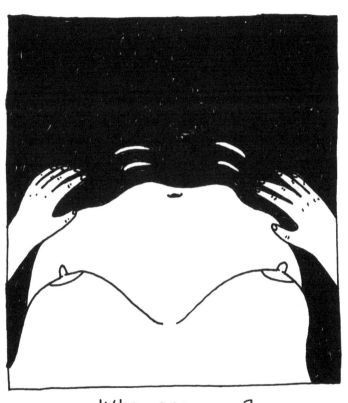

Who are you?

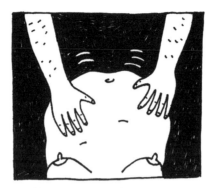

I think my boyfriend
feels jealous.

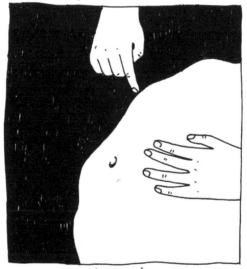

I tell him he's lucky he's
not constantly being kicked
from the inside of his body.

But I also like feeling
your movements.

Sometimes I think that
I will miss carrying you
in my belly.

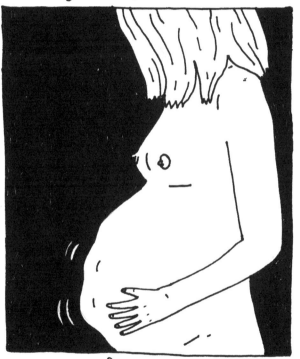

I never feel lonely with
you in there.

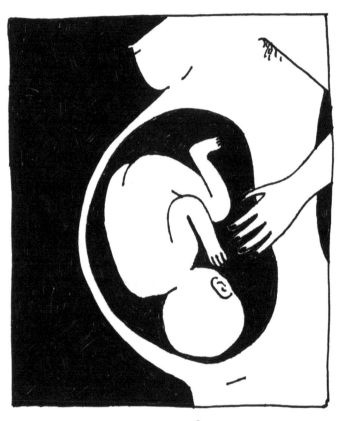

So close but so far away.
Just some skin and liquids
between you and the world.

2.
Questions.

What is the point of having kids?

_____

What is the point of not having kids?

_____

Sometimes I think about the pregnancy that I ended.

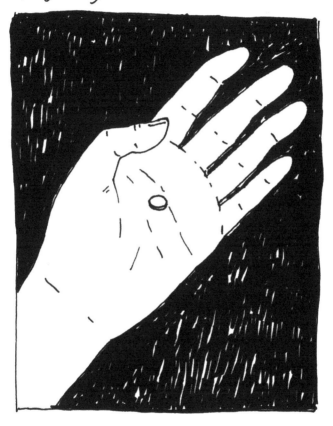

I was grieving after my brother committed suicide, and I could not bring another life into this hard world.

Even now there are so
many things that I
worry about.

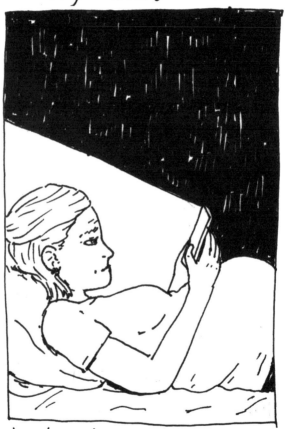

I try to avoid reading
the news.

I made the mistake of reading a book about climate change. and it has given me so much anxiety.

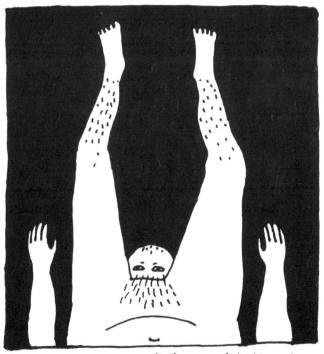

why am I giving birth to a child who has to live on this planet we've fucked up?

WHY ARE YOU MAKING A **BABY**?? WE DON'T NEED MORE HUMANS.

Hey, maybe your life will be easier if you just stay in my warm womb?

A part of me wants to just
stop thinking about the future
and live a happy, wasteful,
ignorant life.

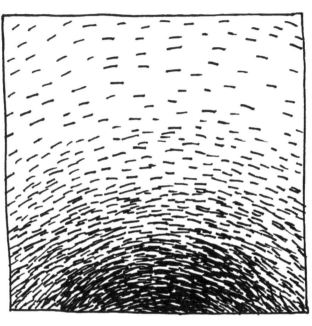

Just ignore the impending doom.

My attitude toward climate
change scares me.

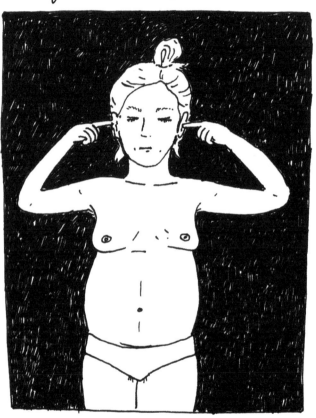

I probably need a car now
that I'm having a baby.

It is hard to have so much choice.

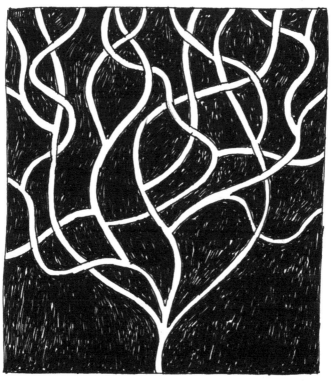

Considering climate change with every decision in life is exhausting.

There is so much focus on my body
right now that I almost forget
that I will have to know what
to do with the baby when
he's born.

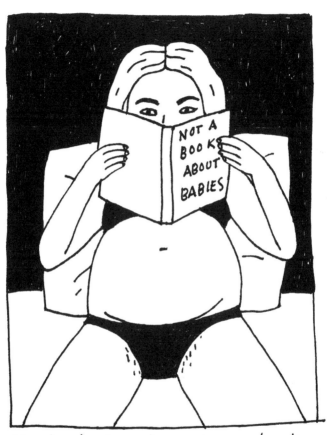

Maybe I should read a book about how to take care of a baby?

People mostly complain
about how hard it is
to have children.
Do they even like being
parents?
Can someone please talk
about the good bits?

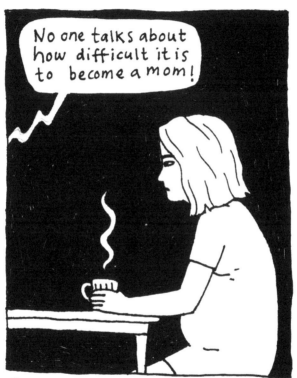

That is all they talk about.

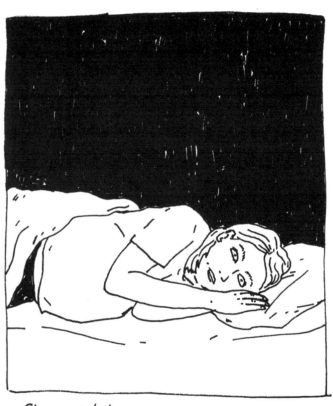

Sleep while you can.

Are you drinking wine when you're pregnant?!
Aren't you having a glass of wine?. You know you can have a drink when you're pregnant.

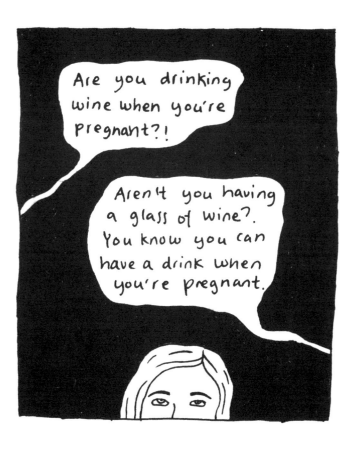

I try to remember that most people have good intentions — even when it feels like they are trying to tell me what to do.

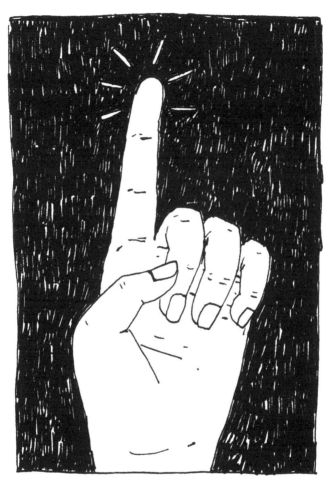

People who give a lot of advice annoy me. But it also annoys me when other mothers complain about getting advice.

When I think about giving birth,
I'm equally terrified and excited.

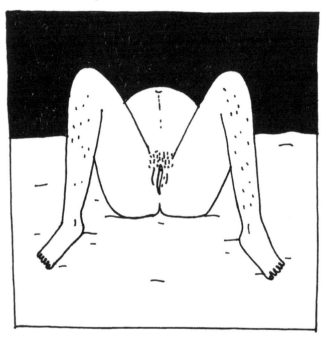

How are you going to get
out of there?!

I'm surprised when my water breaks on the actual due date.

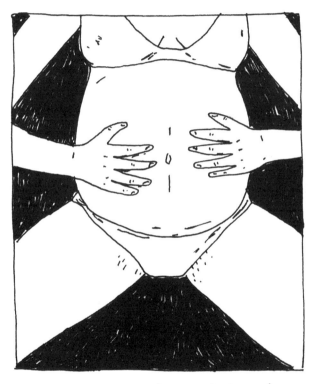

We go to the hospital, and they tell us to go home and wait.

When we go back later at night, my contractions suddenly feel so strong.

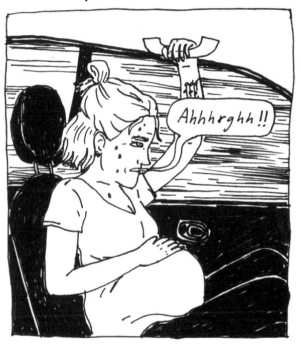

I worry that I might give birth in the car.

When the labor actually starts,
it's a blur. What feels like
an hour is apparently four hours.

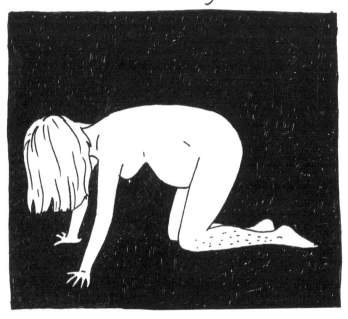

I feel so aware that I am an animal.

I stop responding to the offerings and questions from my partner.

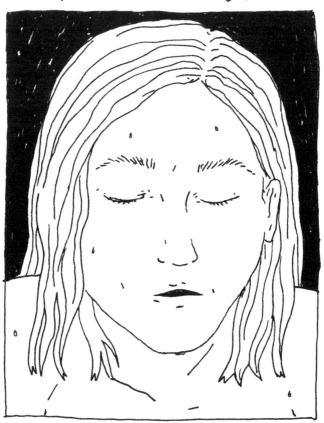

I'm busy breathing.

Throughout pregnancy I have tried to accept that I might not get the birth that I have planned and hoped for.

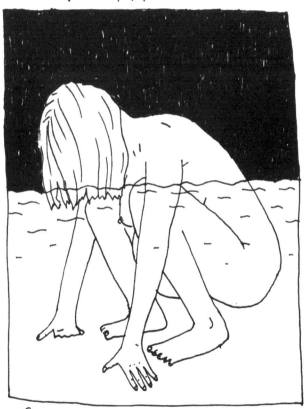

So I'm so grateful that I get to experience a water birth.

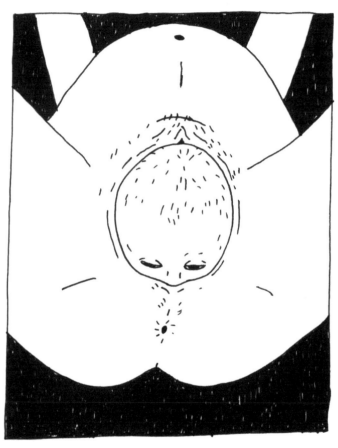

Is it a bit crazy to wish
that I had a photo of
this moment?

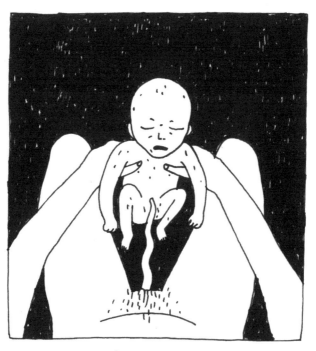

when I first held you.

It is so strange and wonderful
to finally have you on my chest.

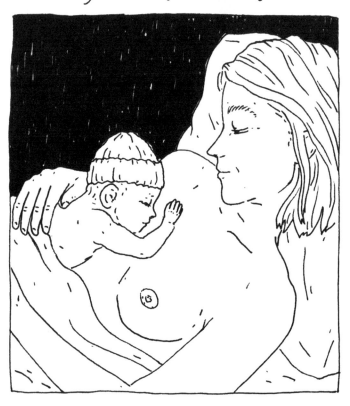

My little boy, skin-to-skin
for the first time.

3.
Milk.

YOUR BODY CREATED A NEW PERSON!

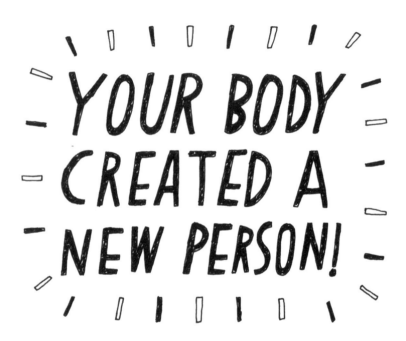

I'm not just fascinated
that I made a little person,
but that other women can
do it too?!

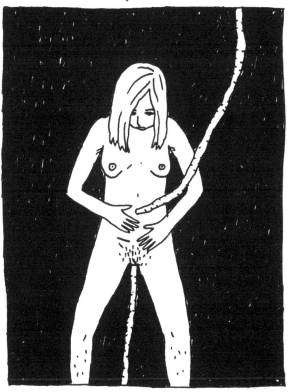

I feel so connected to the
previous generations of mothers.

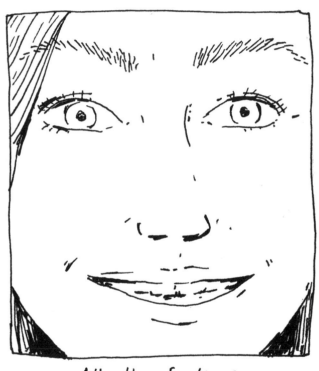

All the feelings.

I don't know what
to do with all the
FEELINGS
you make me feel

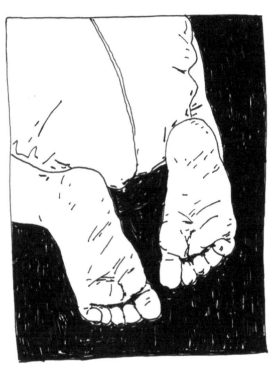

Unused wrinkly feet.
How did I make these?!

How can they
be so small?

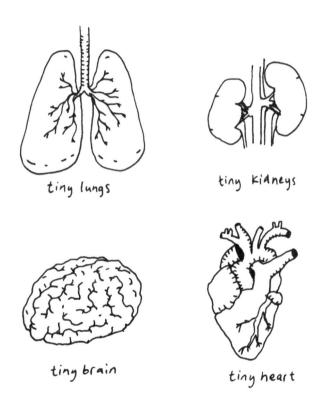

tiny lungs

tiny kidneys

tiny brain

tiny heart

I like to imagine what your
tiny little baby organs look like.

our apartment feels so different
now that we're home with you.

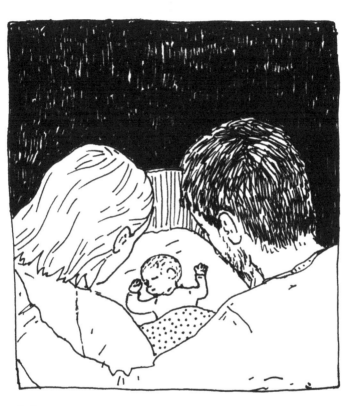

We get to live with this
little person now.

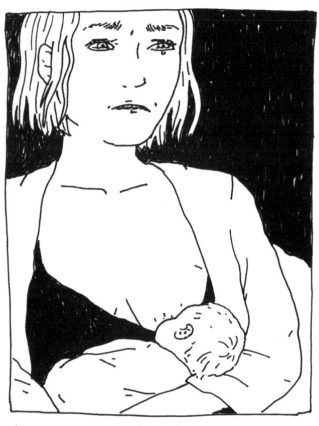

Nursing is hard.

My nipples are sore, and every time I put the baby down he wakes up and starts screaming for more milk.

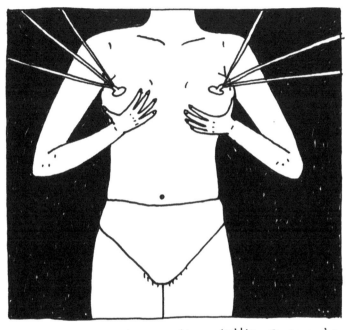

At first, when the milk came in,
I felt like a goddess.

But now, I'm so close to waking
my partner and telling him to
go buy some formula.

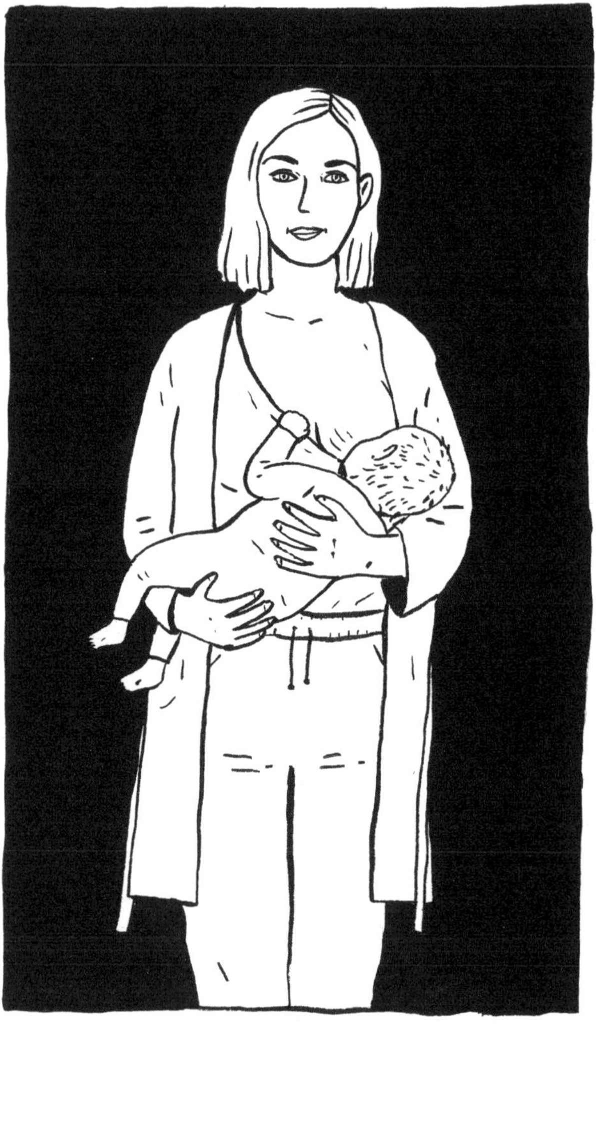

Slowly, we figure out
how to do this.

OXY
TOCIN

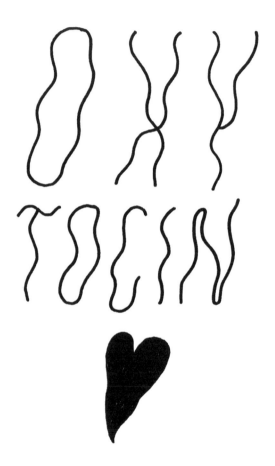

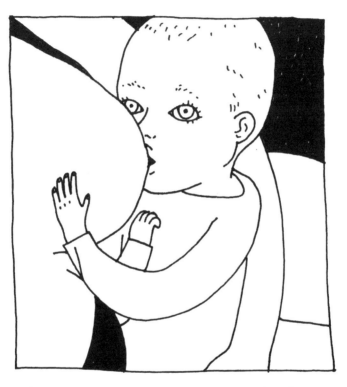

And now I'm addicted.

When can we have
another one?

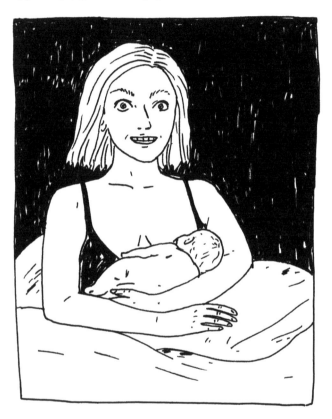

Me, high on hormones.

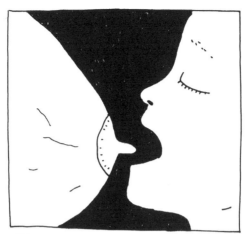

This is normal now.

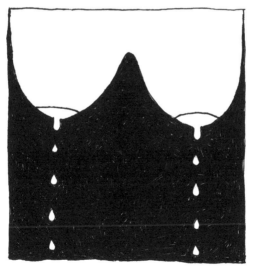

I'm made of food.

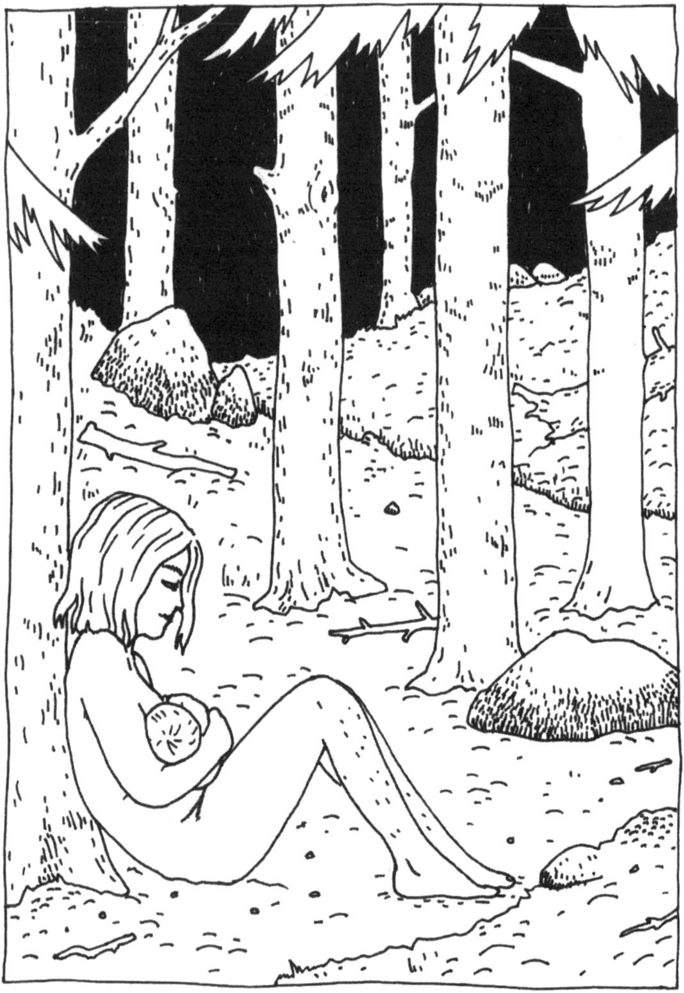

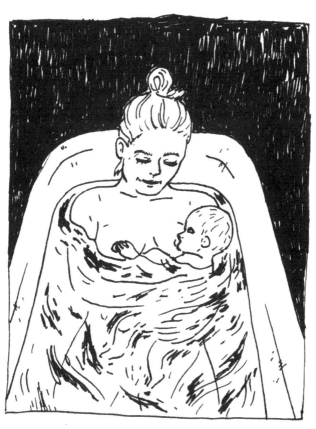

We both love this.

Seeing other animals feed their babies makes me feel so emotional.

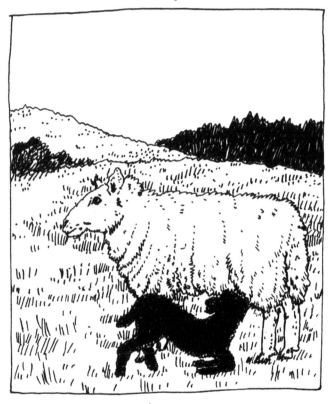

I think about how we, in many ways, are the same.

Get used to seeing my boobs, because I'm not even thinking about covering myself up.

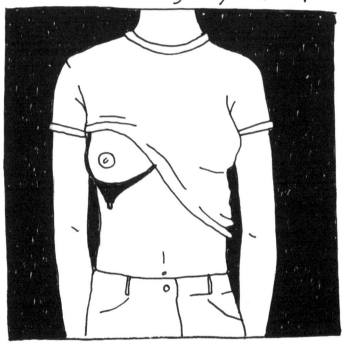

It feels normal to walk around with one boob out.

My baby and I
always want to eat
at the same time.

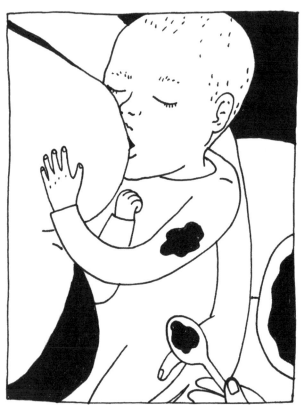

I often spill food on him.

My breasts used to be erotic.

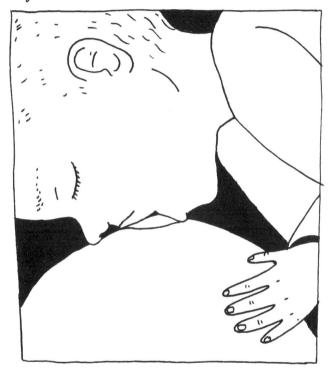

It is pretty weird that my partner used to lick these for fun and now my baby eats from them.

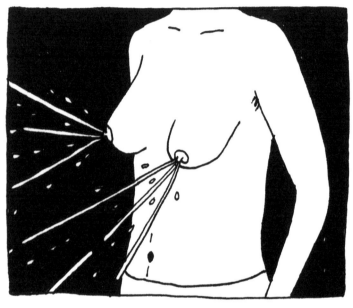

What happens when I don't
wear a bra.

milk

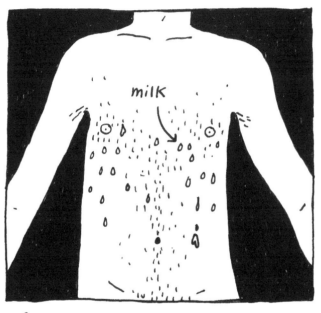

Sexy breast milk spray.

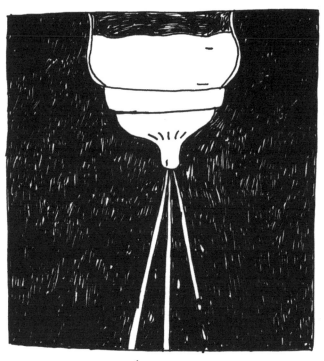

Sometimes, I feel superior to women who choose formula, but I realize that is only because I feel jealous of them.

Breastfeeding is exhausting, and it's frustrating that my partner can't help.

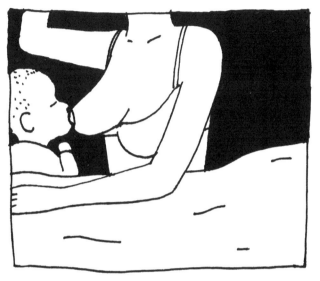

I wish I had longer boobs
so that I could more easily
breastfeed lying down.

AMAZING   BOOBS.

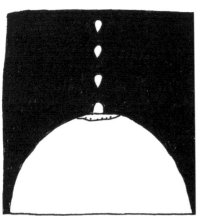

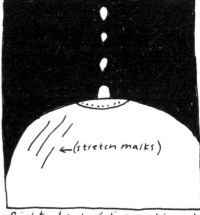

Left boob

Right boob (slightly bigger)

In spite of everything,
I like my breasts more
than I ever have.

4.
Postpartum.

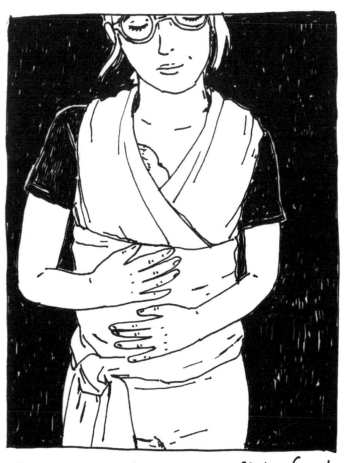

So little that you still feel
like a part of me.

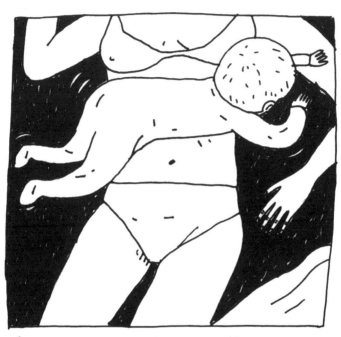

Sometimes I forget that you
came from inside of me!?

It is still weird.

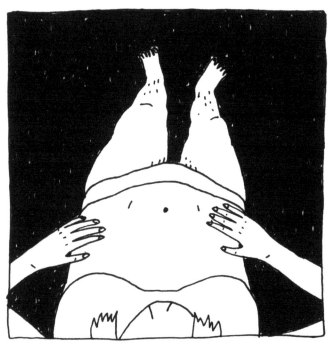

My belly looks different now,
and I realize I don't mind.

I think I like that you can tell
from my body that I carried
a child.

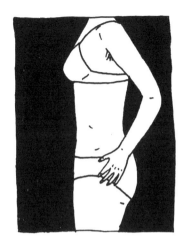

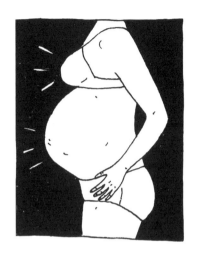

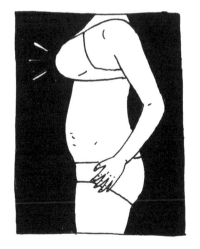

It is pretty amazing
how the belly
can just do that.

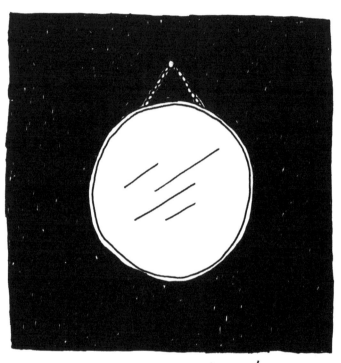

My whole relationship to my
appearance has changed.

Morning/evening routine after becoming a mother.

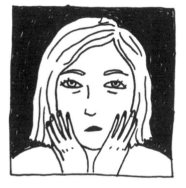

Don't wash face.

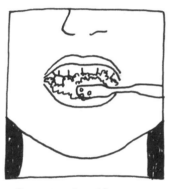

Brush teeth.

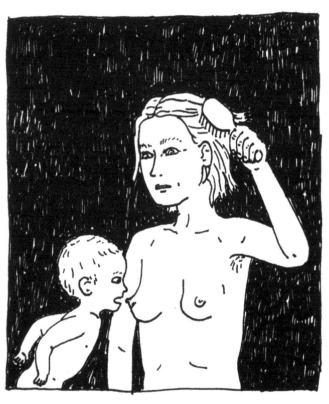

I'm finding these situations equally cute and annoging.

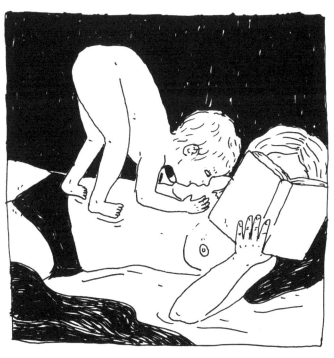

What is so good about
feeding upside down?

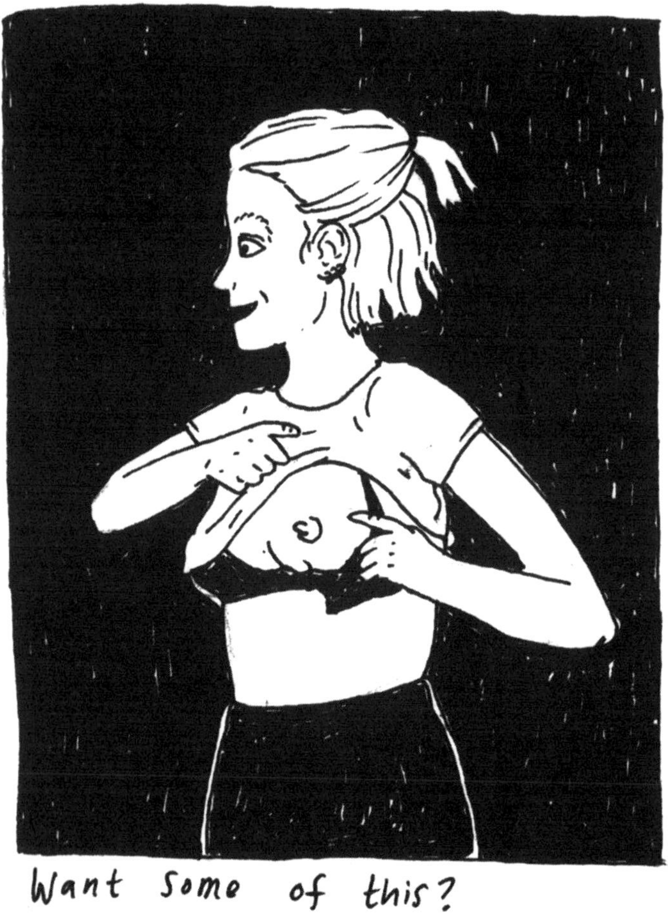

Want some of this?

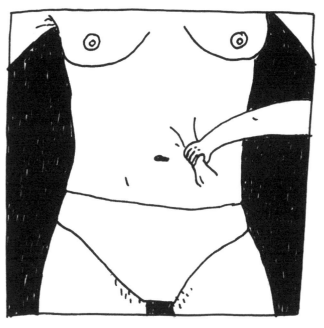

My baby likes to grab the soft skin on my belly.

It is good to have some stretchy soft skin for him to play with.

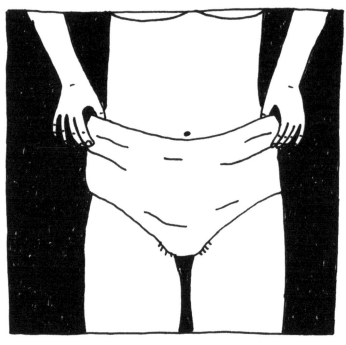

I bought giant underwear to wear after giving birth.
I'm still wearing them because they are so comfy.

I have only now realized
that I have probably been
buying a size too small
for my entire adult life.

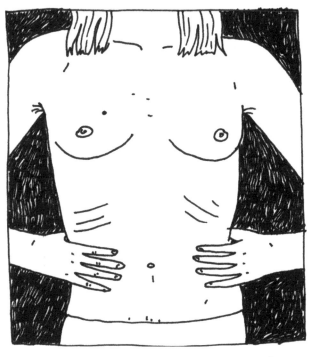

I lost so much weight while breastfeeding that I thought I was seriously ill. I went to see my doctor who told me it was obviously due to stress and breastfeeding.

I was scared of talking
about this because losing
weight is what you are
'meant' to focus on after
giving birth and someone
might just tell me how
lucky I am.

He's getting used to being
bottle fed, by his dad and is
starting to reject my breast.
It makes me feel a bit sad.

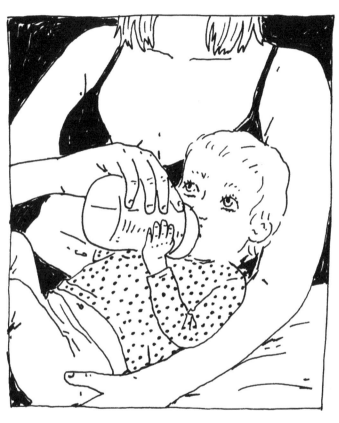

But this is also very cozy.
Sadly, pumping is not.

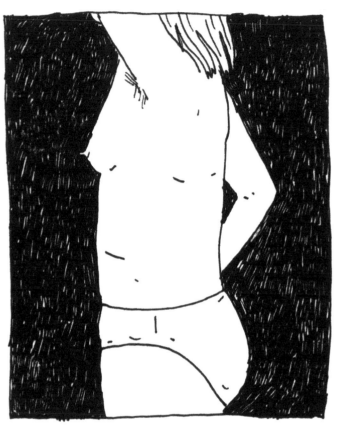

After having gone up in size
while I was breastfeeding,
I hate going back to my
flat chest.

I feel disappointed with myself for not being the kind of person who doesn't care about their breast size.

Useless breasts.

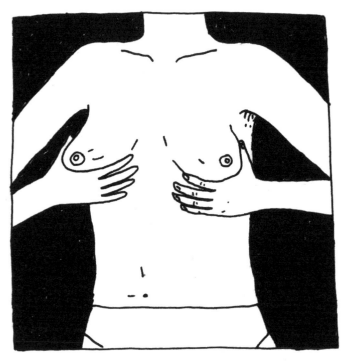

I feel both sad and liberated
that these breasts will
no longer milk.

Post-pregnancy body: I've never felt stronger. I've never felt weaker.

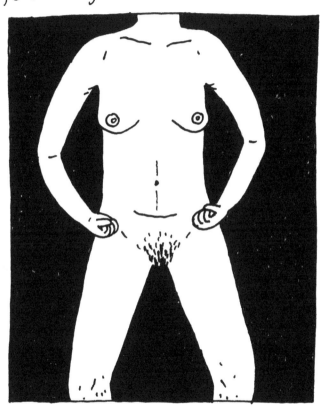

Thanks body. You're pretty great after all.

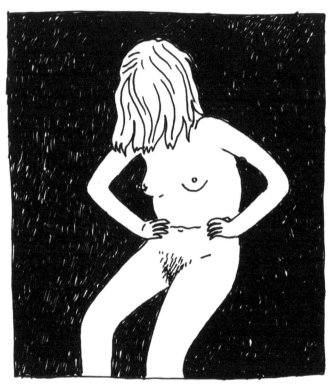

I'm going to live in this
body for the rest of my life.

5.
Someone's Mother.

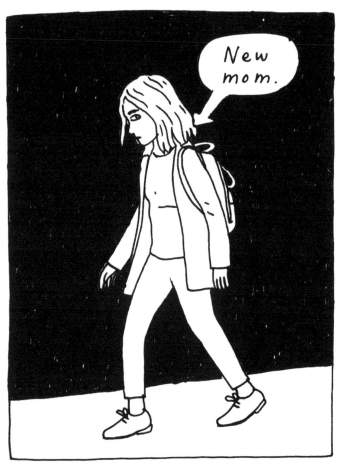

It is the first time I leave my house
without my baby, and it feels so
weird that there are no physical
signs that I'm someone's mother.

Do I look different?
I want everyone to know that
I'm a mother.

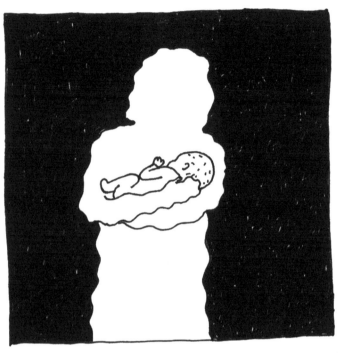

Before I became a mom, I was scared of losing focus on me, but not focusing on me is actually amazing.

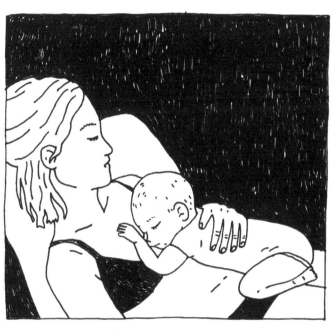

when I feel stressed about
not getting anything done,
I remind myself that cuddling
is very important .

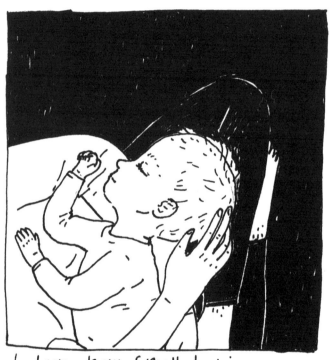

I love how small babies are —
more like little animals than
actual humans.

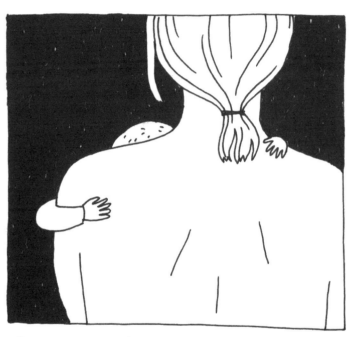

So many hugs.

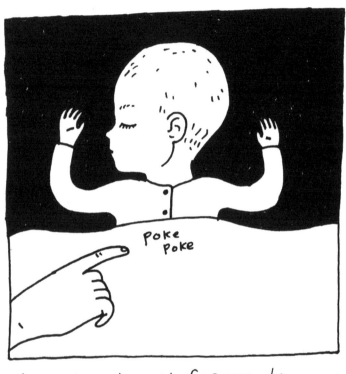

I wait and wait for you to fall asleep, and then I can't wait for you to wake up so that we can hang out.

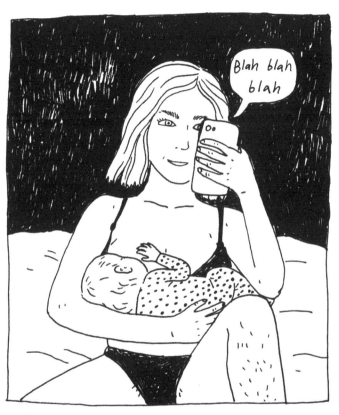

I have never appreciated
smartphones as much as
I do now.

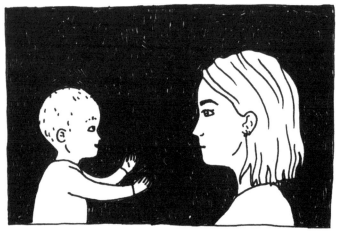

Before I became a mom, I was
worried I might not like babies.

It was hard to know whether
I actually wanted a child or if
it was something that I thought
I wanted because it is the norm.

None of my close friends had children yet, and it was difficult to imagine how amazing it could be.

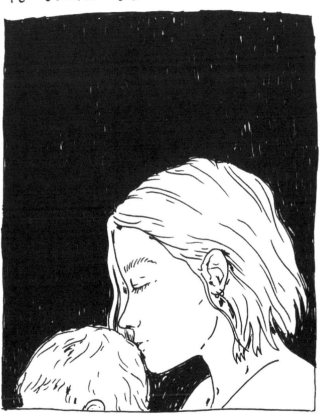

Sometimes I wish I had you sooner.

I STILL DON'T QUITE GET THAT I AM SOMEONE'S

MOM!?

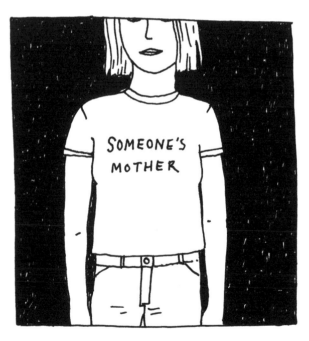

Reminding myself and others.

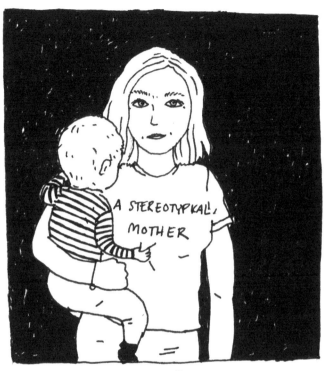

I never used to feel normal, but now it is like I'm becoming a stereotype.

I don't believe in gender roles, but sometimes it feels good to be seen as a mom — whatever that means.

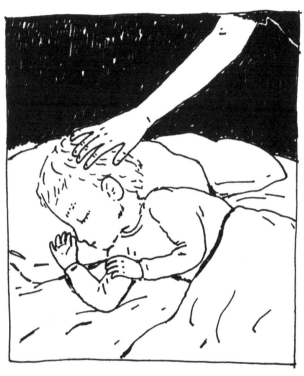

A regular mom who does not
do many extraordinary things
other than being loving,
caring, and supportive.

My main focus at this time of my life is my child, and that is okay. There will be a future where I'll have more time for other parts of my life.

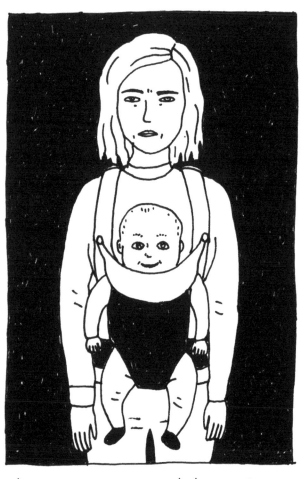

I'm suddenly a lot more approachable.

Somehow, my resting bitch face doesn't work as well now that I have a baby. But it turns out I actually don't hate making small talk with strangers when I can talk about you.

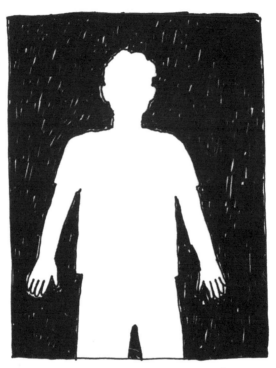

It is both exciting and scary to dream about who you will grow up to be.

What will your interests be? What struggles will you face? What will our relationship be like?

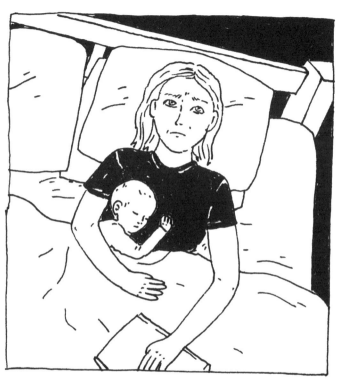

How will climate change
affect you?
Will you be able to dream
about the future?

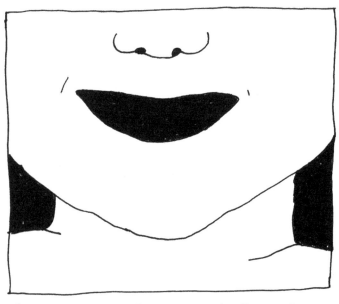

Sometimes when you smile I think
that you're happy now, but you
don't yet know how hard life is.

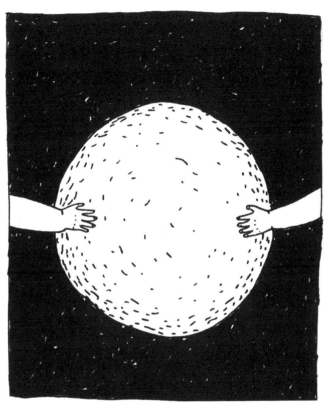

I worry that you will not
be able to create your own
family in this world that
we are destroying.

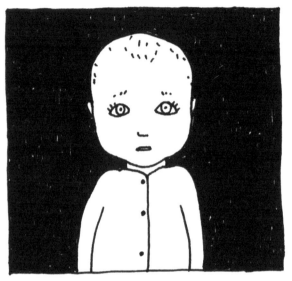

I feel really bad about
ruining this planet for you.

Having a child has
apparently made me
extremely selfish.

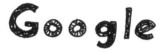

Google

Best country to live climate change X 🔍

My latest Search history.

I think about how
I could live a life that
is not part of this
self-destructive system,
but then I realize how
hard it would be.

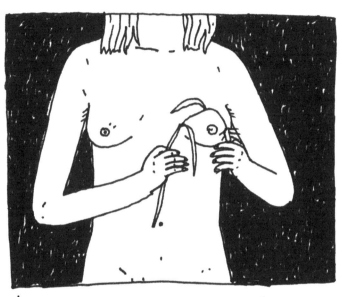

I dream of self-sufficiency,
but who could really survive
on their own in this system?

I'm dreading the day when
I have to tell you about
the severity of climate change.

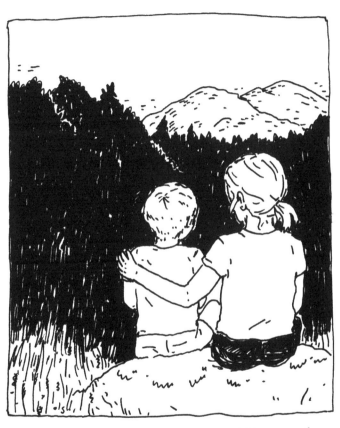

At some point we will need
to have the talk.

When he asks me why
I didn't do anything,
I will think about all
those times I thought about
living a life more true to
myself, but I was too
scared to make a change.

What I will tell my child:

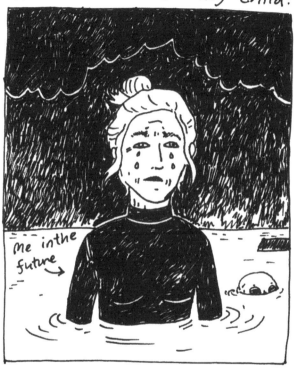

I know we ruined this planet for you, but at least I felt very unhappy while I was doing it.

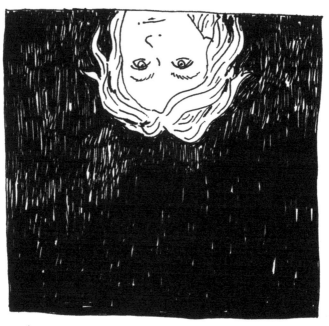

There are so many other
things to worry about too.

It can be overwhelming
at times.

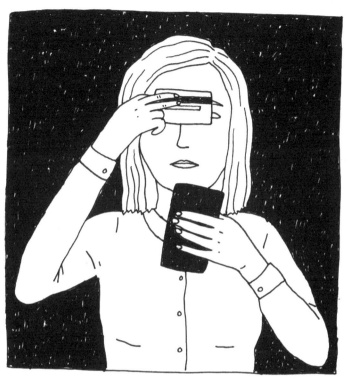

I feel so busy because I need to buy so many things for my family.

Making all of these supposedly essential purchases makes me feel terrible.

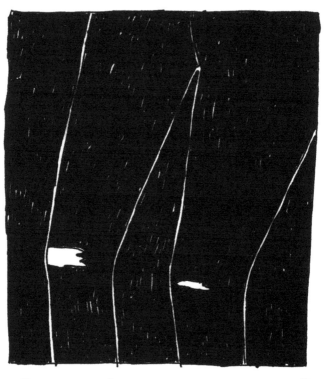

Do I _need_ new yoga leggings?

Mending my clothes again
and again feels like an
act of activism.

The tedious things I do to
stop consuming.

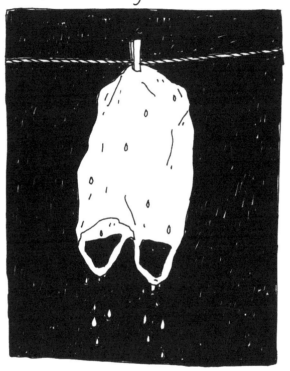

Washing and reusing my plastic
bags may not make a big
difference in the battle against
climate change, but doing even
small things calms my anxiety.

I'm also constantly trying
to get rid of stuff.

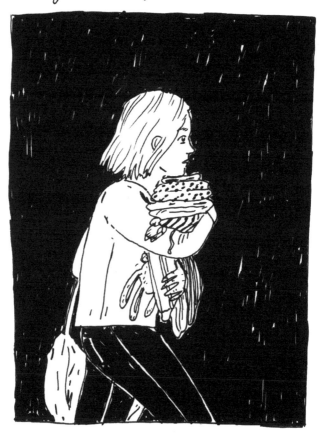

I dream about minimalism,
but what if I need all of
these things one day?

I worry about how I will
make decisions about my future,
Knowing that now, everything
I do impacts you too.

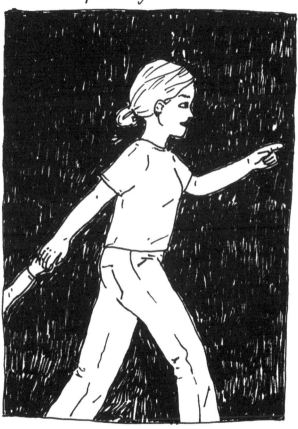

I want to go this way.

This is getting too depressing.

I wanted to talk about how fun it is to be a mother!

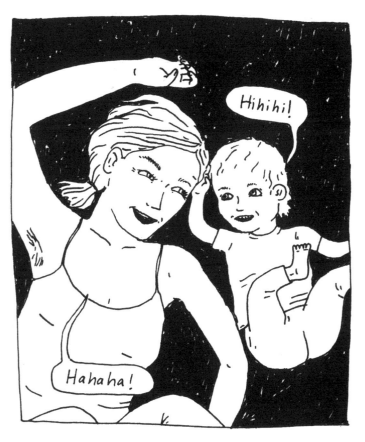

No one told me it would be
so much fun.

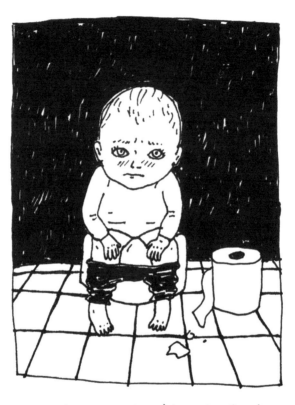

Is it weird that I find my pooping baby one of the cutest things there is?

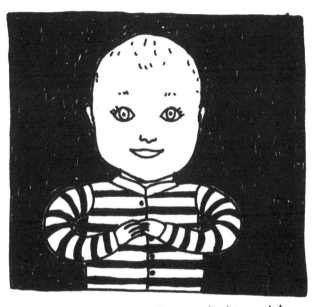

It is completely unbelievable
that you will be an adult
one day, and that ALL
grown-ups were once cute
little babies.

We dance in the kitchen
before breakfast.

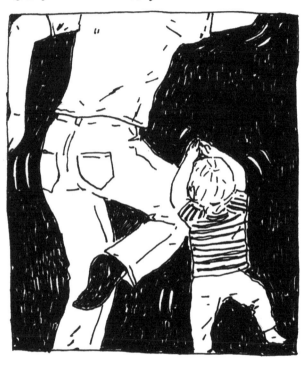

I'm amazed by how he
moves to music.

I laugh more than I used to.

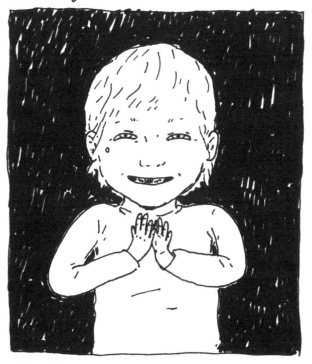

He has already learned how
to make jokes. He laughs out
loud at himself, and it is
hilarious.

I wonder how I will manage
in the future, when I'm expected
to work and have a social life,
as well as be a parent.

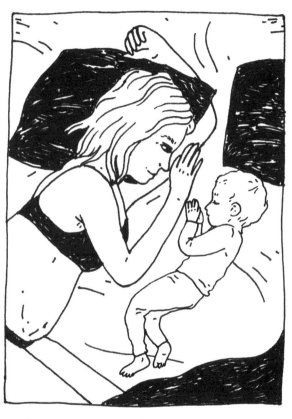

Even when he gets older,
I should allow myself to
relax like this.

When I manage not to be stressed about everything I have to do, I love bedtime.

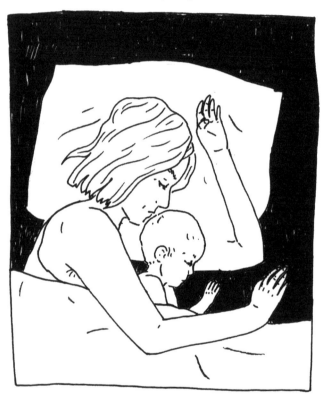

My child could probably fall asleep on his own, but I don't want to miss this.

6.
Equal Parenting.

Built-in inequality.

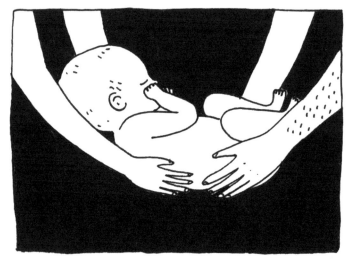

You think it is possible to
live in an equal relationship
with a man, and then you have
a child together.

It turns out that being parents together is hard, even when you have a great relationship.

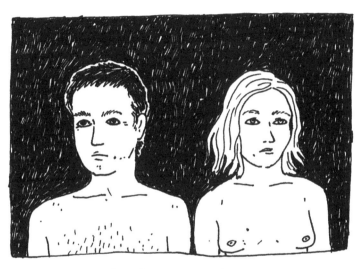

We are both sleep-deprived and sometimes forget to be kind to one another.

It is probably due to
the milk, but it does
feel good that my child
is obsessed with me
right now.

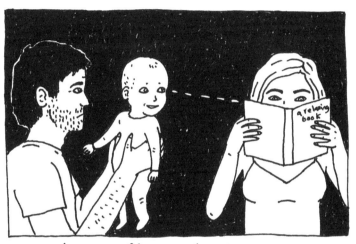

Our baby often only has eyes
for me.

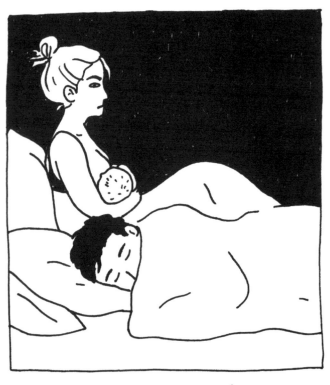

I'm so annoyed at you for sleeping.

I know it makes sense
for him to sleep so that
he can clean and cook
me food tomorrow, but
I just want to wake him
up because it is so lonely
to breastfeed all night.

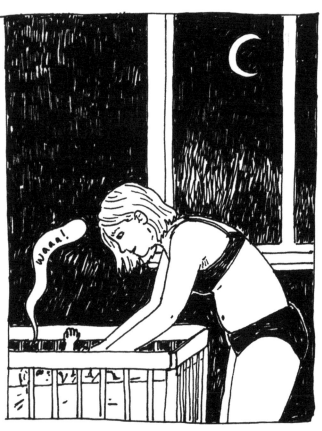

I'm amazed it's possible to
do everything I do with so
little sleep.

The baby always seems to wake up just when I want to have a moment with my partner.

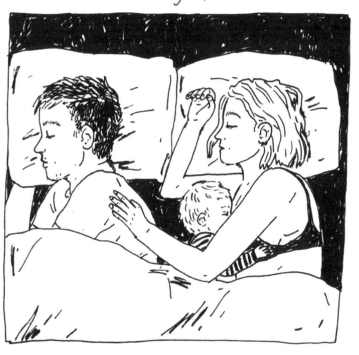

Now we are always three.

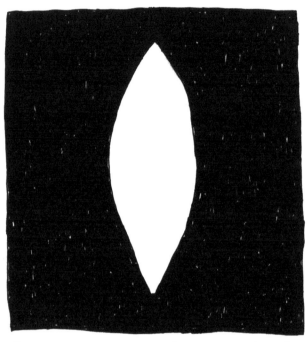

How will I ever feel like having
sex again now that a person
has traveled through my vagina?

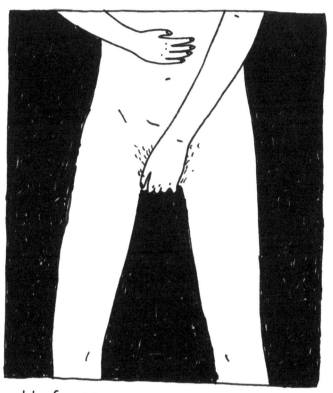

It feels as if it is all
going to fall out.

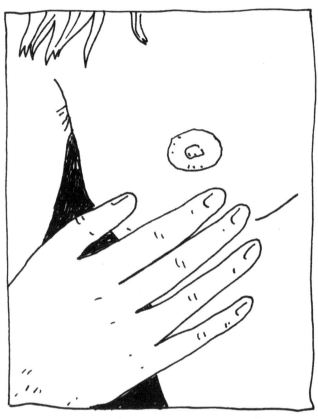

Most days, I feel like I get enough
cuddles from our child.

There is just not enough
time in my day for everyone,
but I miss sex too.

We argue a lot about who does more housework at the moment.

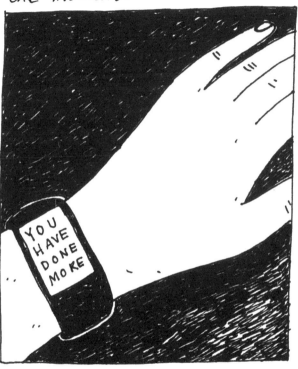

Idea: A smart wristband that tells you exactly how much household and emotional work you've done compared with your partner.

My partner just told me
he is impressed with my
ability to do all the
housework with a baby
by my side.

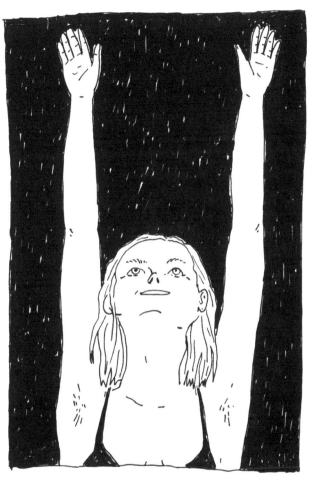

Yes, I'm better than you at multitasking.

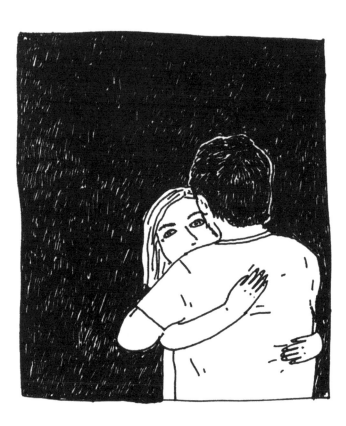

At my most unsympathetic moments, I think that I Should've found a baby daddy with more money.

I care less about money than I ever thought I would, but having a child is expensive.

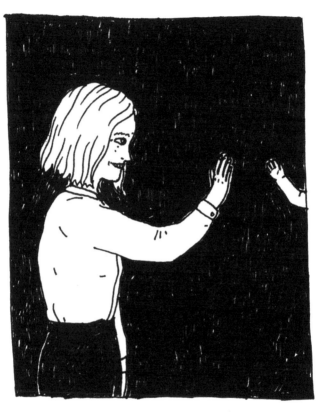

I feel upset with feminism,
because today I'm going back
to work and my partner
will be with our baby.

Even before I got pregnant, I didn't love my job.

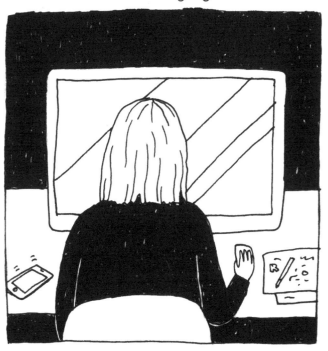

I've heard people say work is a nice break from parenting, but somehow, it doesn't usually feel that way.

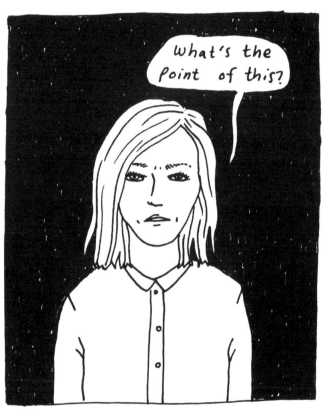

It would all be so much easier if I could just believe in capitalism.

I want to interact with and help people in a meaningful way.

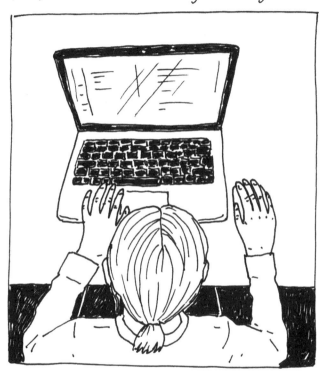

And not spend so much time sending emails and moving pixels.

I feel even more strongly now that I need a job that makes a positive difference in the world.

I would love to get out of the house and work hard at something I care about.

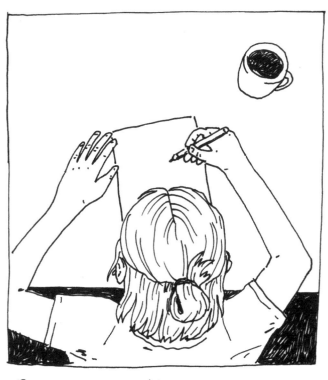

Because sometimes, when I get to work on my art, having a break from my baby feels great.

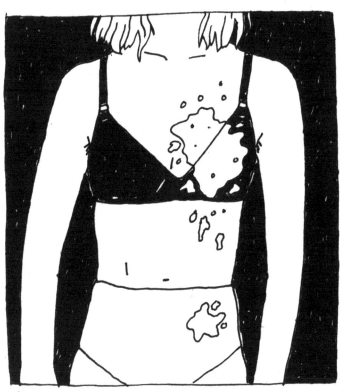

Sometimes it feels more meaningful being at home getting puked on by my child.

It's true that it can be repetitive and overwhelming. But I also find it satisfying to take care of my family and my home.

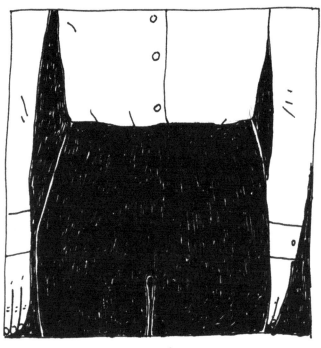

When I'm sitting in a long
meeting at work, at least I
can do some pelvic floor
exercises at the same time.

Can you do too many pelvic
floor exercises?

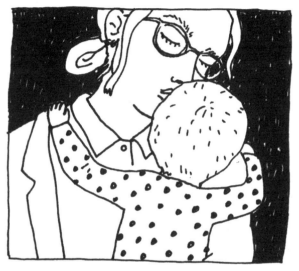

When I say goodbye to you
in the morning, I remind
myself that I'm lucky
to have options.

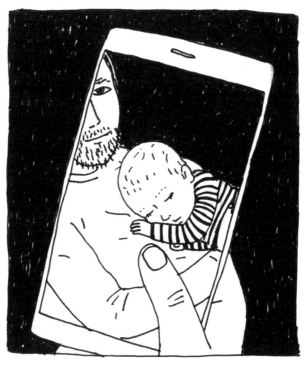

But when I'm at work, I'm so annoyed that you two are at home having fun together.

So sad to be
a feminist.

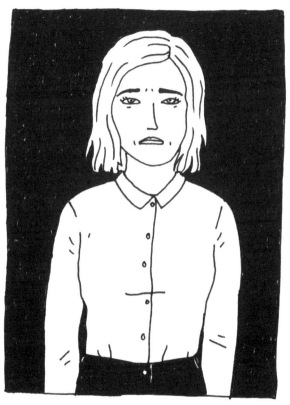

When you want equality but
don't want to share your time
at home with the baby.

When I see how much
you love each other,
I know that sharing
this time was the right
thing to do.

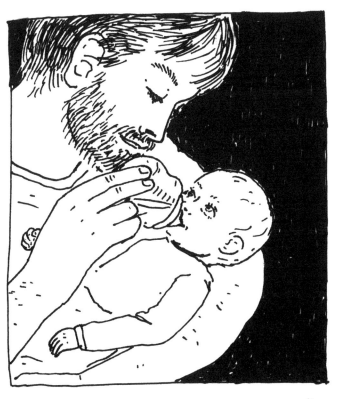

Seeing your partner becoming the best parent is so hot.

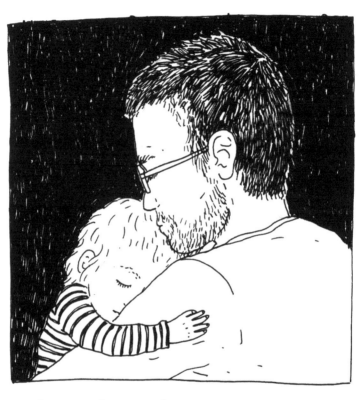

I have been looking forward to
seeing you as a father since
we met. I always knew you
would be a great father.

7.
A mother and
a friend.

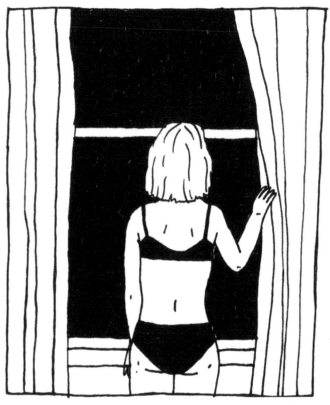

One of the hardest things about having a child is being so far away from my family.

I live in another country from my parents, and sometimes I wish I had never moved.

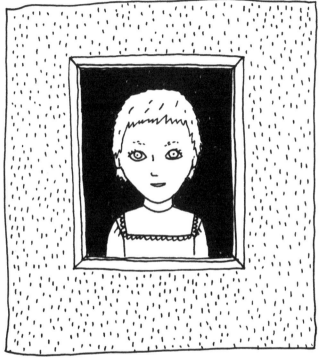

I want to relive my childhood
by giving my child everything
I had when I was growing up.

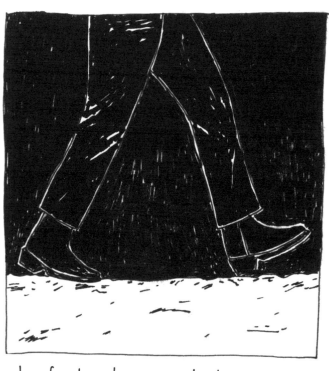

I feel alone, and I am angry at individualism for making me think it was important to pursue my career at the cost of a community.

I'm struggling to have a social life and be a parent at the same time.

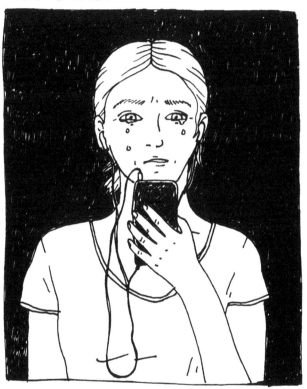

When I try to organize something, it feels like people always have plans for the next four weeks.

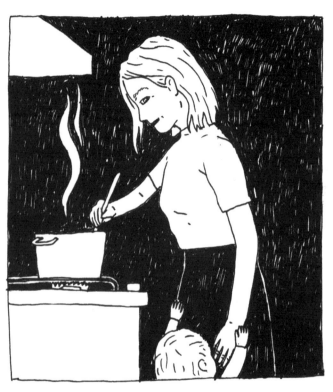

I dream of a commune because
this isolated family life just
doesn't feel like the way
we are meant to live with children.

I want to be more social,
but I don't want to
leave my house very often.

My partner and I are both good at giving each other time to ourselves.

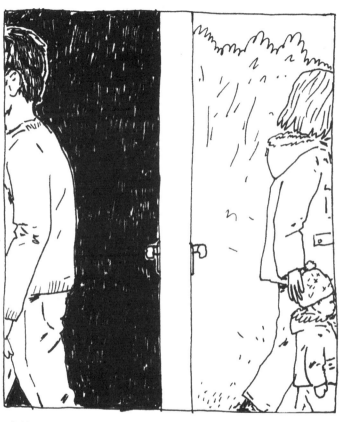

Allowing both of us to have some space sadly means we get less time together as a whole family.

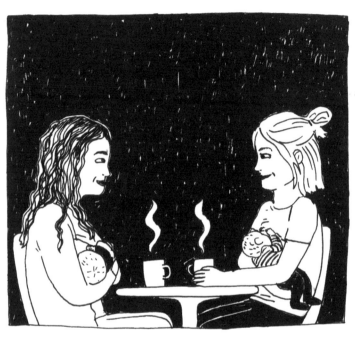

I had too high hopes for how easy it would be to make new mom friends while on maternity leave. I made very few, and I feel lonely.

Is it too picky to want
to have more in common
other than motherhood?

I judge people
who put bows
on their baby girls'
bald heads.

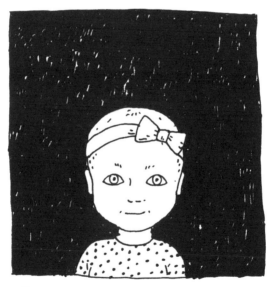

Definitely not a boy.

All baby clothes <u>must</u> have
animal ears.

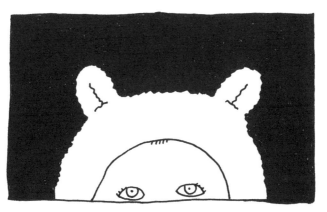

Who came up with this?

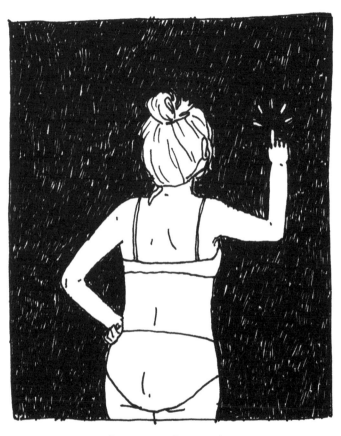

I sometimes feel that I'm
much better at being a mother
than others.

But I also don't want to be
that judgy or self-righteous mom.

It took some time, but eventually, I found mom friends who really got it. Dealing with the hard parts of parenting can be easier when you know you're not the only person struggling.

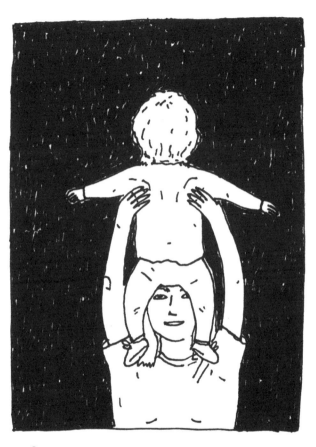

So many other people are
feeling the exact same
feelings right now.

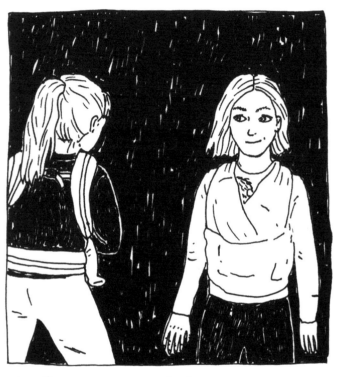

I feel connected to other mothers
I see when I'm out.

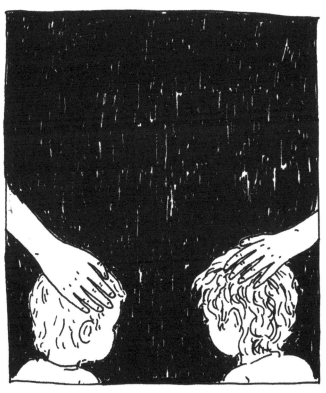

Motherhood can be such a strong force of connection between women, and I love having conversations about being a mom.

Sometimes I just want to talk to my friends, but I'm also excited about getting to know their kids.

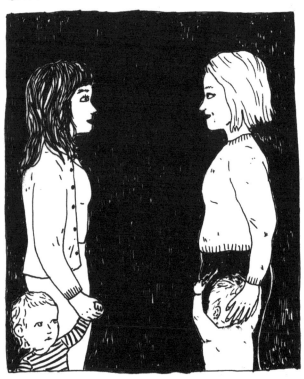

I can't wait to see them grow up and find out what kind of people they will become.

Things I miss as an adult:
Having sleepovers with
my girlfriends.

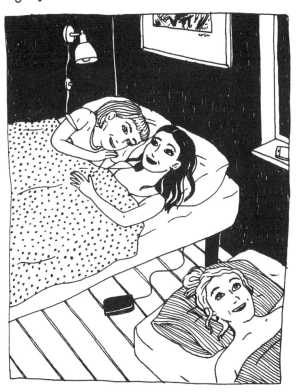

Chatting all night.

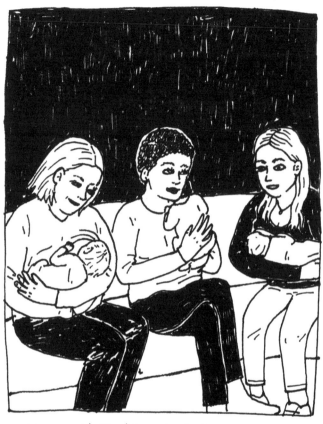

Now, this is what hanging out looks like, and I'm surprised to find that I don't mind.

With my mom friends I feel strong and supported.

8.
A mother and an artist.

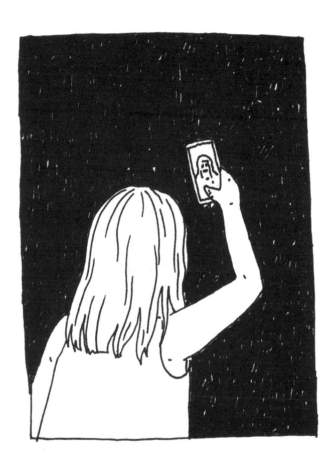

I was going to
draw something NOT
about babies, but
I could not think
of anything.

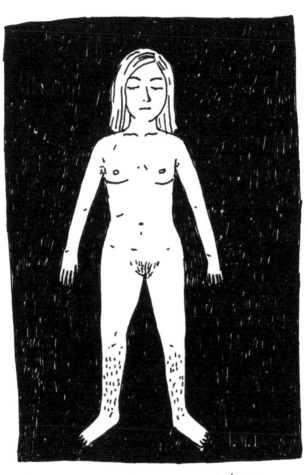

Who am I now when
there are so many things
I no longer care about?

It is not just that I have
no time for lots of things
I used to do before becoming
a parent. I have stopped
even caring about a lot
of things.

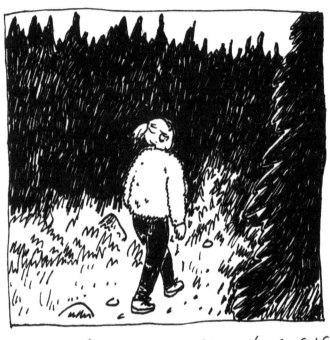

Still, I love having time to myself.

Not having someone clinging to me and having to pack a bag full of baby stuff feels like freedom.

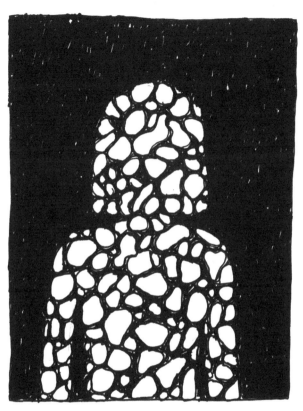

Other times I feel sad because
there are so many parts of me
that I would like to develop,
but there is no time.

How do you choose what not
to do?

– Have you seen that
new TV show?

– No I haven't.

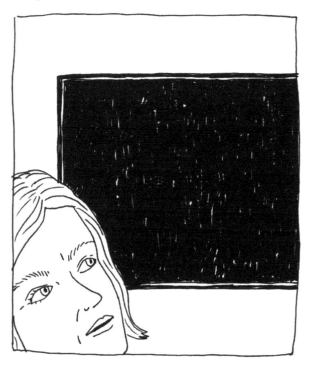

I have no time to watch
TV at the moment, which
means I can't have conversations
with humans.

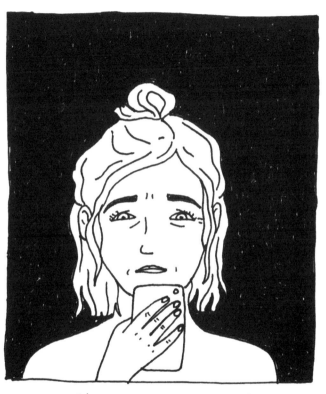

Every time someone unfollows
me, I think it is because I'm
a boring old mom now.

Interesting Mother.

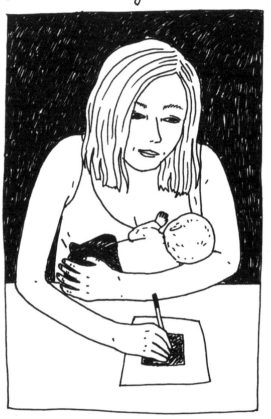

I don't know how to be
an artist and a mother.

For years I have been too scared to ask my employer if I could work part-time to make more time for my art.

Now I can't afford to work less because I have to pay for childcare.

I'm really scared
of becoming a
"mommy blogger" instead
of an artist.

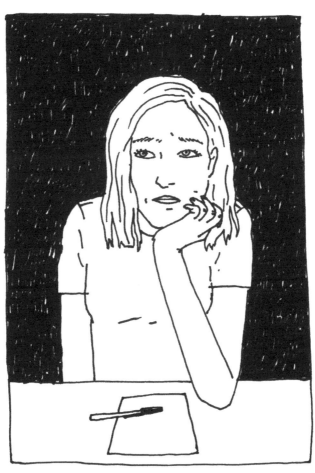

Do I have to change my
username to something with
"mom" in it now?

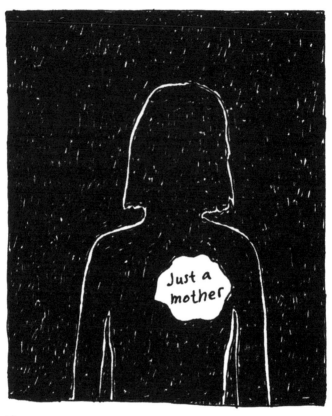

I'm conscious that I do
not want to become someone
who can't talk about anything
except being a mother.

I don't want my child to grow up with the pressure of having a parent who has given up everything in their life for them.

Having limited time has made me realize what I really need in my life, and that is to make art.

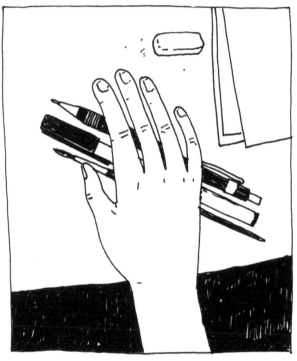

I have become very good at grabbing every moment I can, when I feel inspired.

When I don't have the energy to be creative, I just want to lie down and read a book.

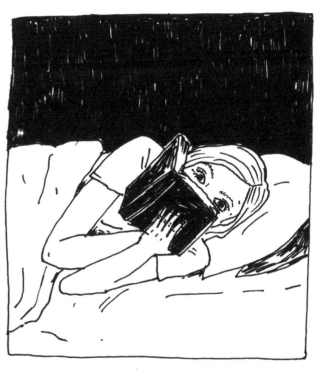

I like not having any weekend plans and not feeling like a failed person.

I never thought I would make a book about having a baby, but when I became a mom it felt like an important thing to do.

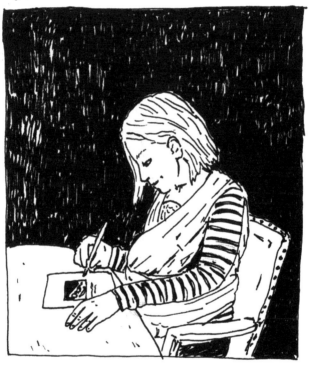

Motherhood as a subject has opened up to me, and I love exploring it in my art.

9.
Can we have another one?

It is hard to imagine what life was like before.

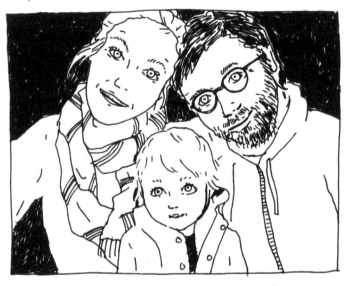

I love having a little family.

The excitement when I've been focusing on work all day and remember I get to go and hang out with my kid soon.

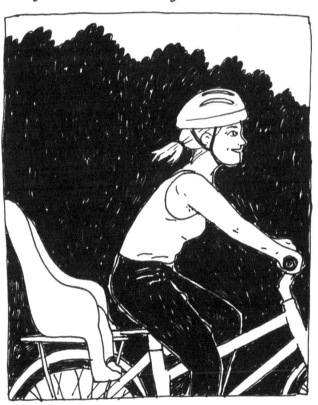

I love that I have someone that I can miss this much.

There are lots of things that I wish I had recorded better as I only now realize how easy it is to forget, as we constantly form new memories together.

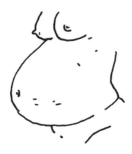

The pregnancy

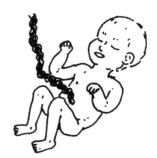

The birth

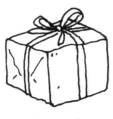

Presents

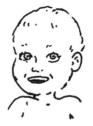

First smile

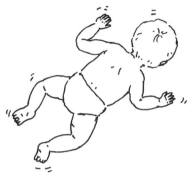

First time rolling over

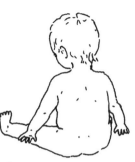

First time sitting up

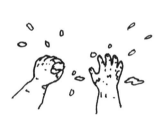

First foods

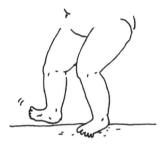

First Steps

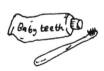

First tooth

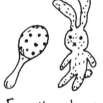

Favorite toys

Everything was new and special.

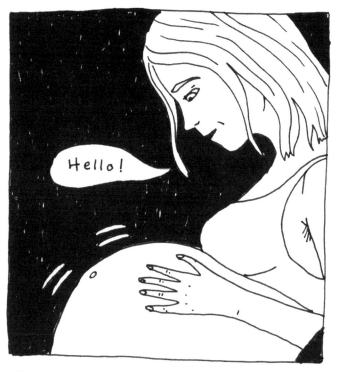

Sometimes I feel sad that I won't experience having my first child again.

How did it happen?

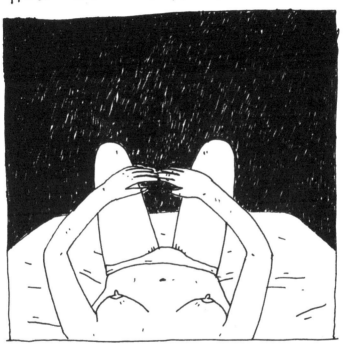

I try to remember exactly what it was like to be pregnant.

I might get addicted to
making babies now.

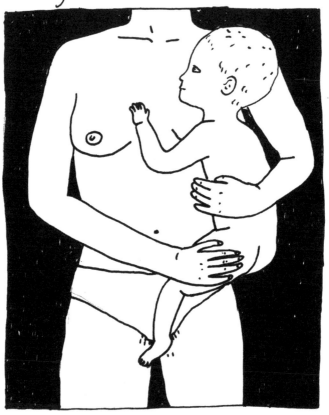

Even if my body has done it once,
I find it unbelievable that it could
possibly make another human one day.

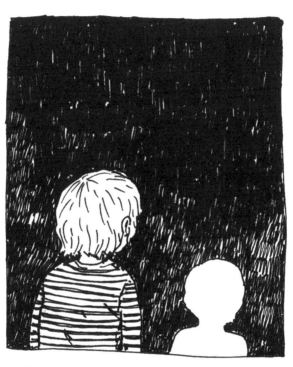

If we do it again, it will be an entirely different human with their own unique personality.

But right now I am busy
experiencing this.

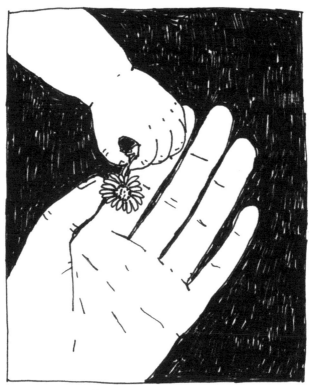

Mommy flower.

Things that were boring
are suddenly fun again.

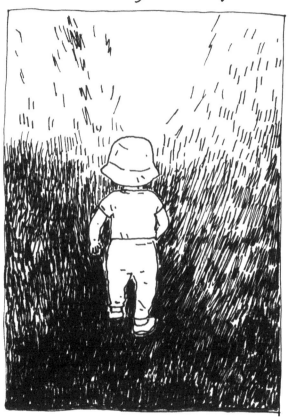

Seeing the world through
your eyes.

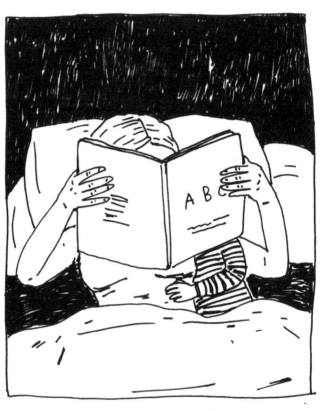

We're going to read thousands of books together.

And teach each other
lots of things.

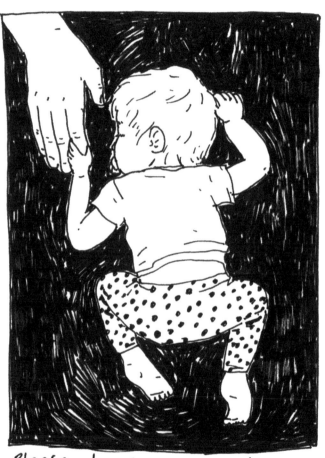

Please don't grow up too quickly.

Acknowledgments

First of all I want to thank my partner Gordon for all your love, support, and for giving me two beautiful children. It is very true that this book would never have been if it were not for you, or them. Thank you to my son, Tor, and daughter, Runa, for teaching me how to be a mother—it is the best thing that has happened to me. A big thanks to my amazing editor Kristen Hewitt and the team at Princeton Architectural Press, who made this into an actual book.

Thank you to my fantastic agent Maggie Cooper for believing in me and helping me get this book published.

A very special thanks to my best friend Ida Gunnarsson and all our long calls where I get to chat about motherhood, literature, and life.

As this book is about parenthood, I am eternally grateful to my mother, Agnetha, and father, Anders, who made sure my siblings and I had a loving and safe childhood, full of adventure. I want to give my children everything you gave me, which is proof you did a very good job. Thank you to my sisters, Martina and Jenny, for always being there for me. To my brother Henrik for all the fun we had growing up—I wish you could have met your niece and nephew before you left us.

Finally, I could not have made this book without the encouragement and support of my online community. Thank you.

Published by
Princeton Architectural Press
70 West 36th Street
New York, NY 10018
www.papress.com

Editor: Kristen Hewitt
Cover design: Paul Wagner and Emma Ahlqvist

Library of Congress Control Number: 2022933703